GLOBAL CLINICAL TRIALS

Ethics, Regulations, and Best Practices

Dr Essam Abdelhakim

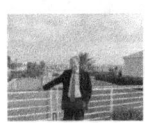

Copyright © 2024 Dr Essam Abdelhakim

All rights reserved

The characters and events portrayed in this book are fictitious. Any similarity to real persons, living or dead, is coincidental and not intended by the author.

No part of this book may be reproduced, or stored in a retrieval system, or transmitted in any form or by any means, electronic, mechanical, photocopying, recording, or otherwise, without express written permission of the publisher.

Cover design by: Art Painter
Library of Congress Control Number: 2018675309
Printed in the United States of America

CONTENTS

Title Page
Copyright
Global Clinical Trials: A Comprehensive Guide for Researchers | 1
Importance of Global Clinical Trials | 2
Understanding Clinical Trial Regulatory Frameworks | 8
Ethical Principles in Clinical Trials | 19
Ethical Challenges in Vulnerable Populations | 23
Differences in Clinical Trial Regulations Globally | 27
Navigating Approvals in Emerging Markets | 30
Ensuring Ethical Conduct in Developing Countries | 34
Case Studies in Multi-Regional Clinical Trials | 36
Practical Strategies for Managing Multi-Regional Trials | 39
Future of Global Clinical Trials | 42
Appendices | 44
About The Author | 47

GLOBAL CLINICAL TRIALS: A COMPREHENSIVE GUIDE FOR RESEARCHERS

Introduction

Clinical trials are the cornerstone of medical research, providing crucial evidence for the safety and efficacy of new treatments.
In an increasingly globalized world, conducting clinical trials across multiple countries and regions has become both a necessity and an opportunity.

This book aims to provide researchers with a comprehensive understanding of the complex landscape of global clinical trials, focusing on regulatory frameworks, ethical considerations, and practical strategies for successful implementation.

The landscape of clinical research has evolved dramatically over the past few decades. What was once primarily a localized endeavor, often confined to a single country or region, has now become a global enterprise.

This shift has been driven by several factors, including:

IMPORTANCE OF GLOBAL CLINICAL TRIALS

Global clinical trials offer several significant advantages that make them an attractive option for researchers and sponsors:

1. Increased Patient Recruitment and Diversity

One of the primary benefits of conducting trials across multiple countries is the ability to access a larger and more diverse patient population.

This is particularly crucial for:

By including participants from various geographical regions, researchers can:

2. Faster Completion of Studies

Global trials can significantly reduce the time required to complete a study by:

This acceleration can lead to:

3. Cost-effectiveness

While global trials can involve higher upfront costs due to the complexity of multi-site coordination, they often prove more cost-effective in the long run.

This is achieved through:

Researchers should conduct thorough cost-benefit analyses that consider both short-term expenses and long-term returns when planning global trials.

4. Broader Applicability of Results

By including diverse populations, global trials can:

This broader applicability can:

5. Access to Expertise and Facilities Worldwide

Global trials allow researchers to:

This global collaboration can:

However, global clinical trials also present unique challenges that researchers must be prepared to address:

1. Navigating Diverse Regulatory Environments

Each country has its own regulatory framework for clinical trials, which can vary significantly in terms of:

Researchers must develop strategies to:

2. Ensuring Ethical Consistency Across Cultures

Ethical standards and practices can vary across cultures, presenting challenges in:

Researchers must strive to:

3. Managing Logistical Complexities

The operational aspects of global trials can be daunting, involving:

Effective management requires:

4. Harmonizing Data Collection and Analysis

Ensuring data consistency and quality across diverse settings is crucial.

Challenges include:

Strategies to address these challenges include:

By understanding both the advantages and challenges of global clinical trials, researchers can better prepare for the complexities involved and develop strategies to maximize the benefits while mitigating potential risks.

Balancing Innovation, Regulation, and Ethics

The conduct of global clinical trials requires a delicate balance between promoting scientific innovation, adhering to regulatory requirements, and upholding ethical standards.

This balance is crucial for ensuring that research is not only scientifically rigorous and compliant but also morally sound and beneficial to society.

Promoting Scientific Innovation

Innovation in clinical trials is essential for advancing medical knowledge and developing new treatments.

Key Aspects Include:

Novel Trial Designs

Innovative Technologies

Biomarker Development

Researchers must:

Adhering to Regulatory Requirements

Regulatory compliance is non-negotiable in clinical research.

Key considerations include:

Understanding Global Regulatory Landscapes

Robust Quality Management Systems

Proactive Regulatory Engagement

Researchers should:

Upholding Ethical Standards

Ethical conduct is paramount in clinical research to protect participants and maintain public trust.

Key elements include:

Informed Consent

Fair Participant Selection

Risk Minimization

Benefit Sharing

Researchers must:

Strategies for Balancing Competing Priorities

Achieving a balance between innovation, regulation, and ethics requires:

1. Integrated Planning
2. Stakeholder Engagement
3. Flexibility and Adaptability
4. Transparent Communication
5. Continuous Education and Training
6. Regular Review and Assessment
   - Conduct periodic reviews of trial

progress to ensure ongoing alignment with regulatory and ethical standards

- Be prepared to make adjustments if imbalances are identified

UNDERSTANDING CLINICAL TRIAL REGULATORY FRAMEWORKS

United States: The Role of the FDA

The U.S. Food and Drug Administration (FDA) plays a pivotal role in overseeing clinical trials conducted in the United States. Understanding the FDA's regulatory framework is crucial for researchers planning to conduct trials in the U.S. or seeking FDA approval for their products.

Investigational New Drug (IND) Application Process

The IND application is a critical step in initiating clinical trials for a new drug in the U.S.

This process involves several key components:

1. Pre-IND Consultation
2. IND Submission
    - Form FDA 1571 (IND application cover sheet)
        - Includes general information about the sponsor, investigators, and study
    - Form FDA 1572 (Statement of Investigator)

- Commitment by investigators to comply with FDA regulations

3. IND Review Process
4. IND Maintenance

Researchers should:

Phases of Clinical Trials and FDA Oversight

The FDA recognizes four primary phases of clinical trials, each with specific objectives and regulatory considerations:

1. Phase I
2. Phase II
3. Phase III
4. Phase IV (Post-Marketing)

For each phase, researchers must:

Key Guidelines: CFR Title 21 and ICH-GCP

Two primary sets of guidelines govern clinical trials in the U.S.:

1. Code of Federal Regulations (CFR) Title 21
   - Part 11: Electronic Records and Electronic

- Signatures
  - Requirements for using electronic systems in clinical trials
- Part 50: Protection of Human Subjects
  - Informed consent requirements and ethical considerations
- Part 54: Financial Disclosure by Clinical Investigators
  - Reporting of financial interests that may introduce bias
- Part 56: Institutional Review Boards
  - Requirements for ethical review of clinical trials
- Part 312: Investigational New Drug Application
  - Detailed regulations on the IND process and conduct of clinical trials
- Part 314: Applications for FDA Approval to Market a New Drug
  - Requirements for New Drug Applications (NDAs)

Researchers must:
While ICH-GCP is not legally binding in the U.S., the FDA strongly encourages adherence to these guidelines.

Researchers should:

European Union: EMA and National Agencies

The regulatory landscape for clinical trials in the European Union (EU) is complex, involving both centralized and national processes.

The European Medicines Agency (EMA) plays a central role in coordinating the evaluation and monitoring of clinical trials across the EU, while national competent authorities retain significant responsibilities.

The Clinical Trials Regulation (CTR) and the European Medicines Agency

The Clinical Trials Regulation (EU) No 536/2014 (CTR) came into effect on January 31, 2022, replacing the previous Clinical Trials Directive.

This regulation aims to harmonize the assessment and supervision processes for clinical trials throughout the EU.

Key features include:

1. Single Application Portal: The Clinical Trials Information System (CTIS)
2. Harmonized Assessment Procedure (continued)
3. Increased Transparency
4. Risk-Adapted Approach
5. Enhanced Safety Reporting

Researchers conducting trials in the EU must:

Harmonization under ICH-GCP

The EU, like many global regions, adheres to the International Conference on Harmonisation Good Clinical Practice (ICH-GCP) guidelines.

Key aspects include:

1. Integration with EU Regulations
2. Specific EU Adaptations
3. Continuous Updates

Researchers should:

Differences Among EU Member States

Despite efforts towards harmonization, some differences in national requirements persist:

1. Ethics Committee Processes
2. Language Requirements
3. Insurance and Liability
4. Data Protection
    - While the General Data Protection Regulation (GDPR) applies EU-wide, its implementation in clinical research contexts can vary
5. Additional National Requirements

Strategies for managing these differences include:

United Kingdom: MHRA Post-Brexit

The United Kingdom's exit from the European Union (Brexit) has led to significant changes in its clinical trial regulatory landscape.

The Medicines and Healthcare products Regulatory Agency (MHRA) now operates independently of the European Medicines Agency (EMA).

Changes in Regulation after Brexit

1. Separate Regulatory System
2. UK Clinical Trials Regulation
3. MHRA as Central Authority
4. Data Acceptance and Recognition
5. Changes in Reporting Requirements

MHRA Approval Processes

The MHRA has streamlined its approval process to maintain the UK's attractiveness for clinical research:

1. Combined Review Service
2. Accelerated Timelines
3. Innovation Passport and Innovative Licensing and Access Pathway (ILAP)
    - New designation for promising medicines that can benefit from accelerated development and review
4. Early Access to Medicines Scheme (EAMS)

- Provides a route for unlicensed medicines to be used in UK clinical practice

5. Risk-Adapted Approaches

Researchers planning trials in the UK should:

Other Regions

Japan: PMDA Guidelines

The Pharmaceuticals and Medical Devices Agency (PMDA) oversees clinical trials in Japan. Key aspects include:

1. Regulatory Framework
2. Clinical Trial Notification (CTN) System
3. Foreign Data Acceptance
4. Local Clinical Trial Requirements
5. GCP Inspections
   - PMDA conducts rigorous GCP inspections, including for foreign sites used in Japanese submissions

Researchers should:

Canada: Health Canada Oversight

Health Canada regulates clinical trials through its Clinical Trials Regulation, which aligns closely with ICH-GCP guidelines:

1. Clinical Trial Application (CTA) Process
2. Research Ethics Board (REB) Approval
3. Good Clinical Practices
4. Safety Reporting
5. Special Access Program
   - Mechanism for accessing unapproved drugs

for patients with serious or life-threatening conditions

Researchers conducting trials in Canada must:

Australia: TGA Framework

The Therapeutic Goods Administration (TGA) regulates clinical trials in Australia, with a focus on streamlined processes:

1. Clinical Trial Notification (CTN) Scheme
2. Clinical Trial Approval (CTA) Scheme
3. Good Clinical Practice (GCP) Inspections
4. Expedited Pathways
   - Priority Review and Provisional Approval pathways for promising new medicines
5. Clinical Trial Exemption (CTX) Scheme
   - Allows supply of unapproved therapeutic goods for use in clinical trials

Researchers should:

India: CDSCO Approval Process

The Central Drugs Standard Control Organization (CDSCO) oversees clinical trials in India. Recent reforms have aimed at improving efficiency and ethical standards:

1. New Drugs and Clinical Trials Rules, 2019
2. Ethics Committee Registration

3. Clinical Trial Registry
   - Mandatory registration of all clinical trials on the Clinical Trials Registry-India (CTRI)
4. Compensation Guidelines
5. Local Clinical Trial Requirements
6. Audio-Visual Recording of Informed Consent
   - Mandatory for vulnerable subjects in clinical trials of new chemical entities

Researchers planning trials in India should:

China: NMPA Regulations

The National Medical Products Administration (NMPA) regulates clinical trials in China, with an increasing focus on aligning with international standards:

1. Drug Registration Regulation (DRR)
2. Good Clinical Practice
3. Human Genetic Resources Regulations
4. Clinical Trial Authorization (CTA) Process
5. Ethics Committee System
6. Data Acceptance

Researchers conducting trials in China must:
- Plan for potentially longer timelines due to complex regulatory processes

- Carefully consider human genetic resource regulations when planning sample collection
- Engage with experienced local partners familiar with NMPA requirements
- Stay informed about rapidly evolving regulations and guidelines

ETHICAL PRINCIPLES IN CLINICAL TRIALS

The Belmont Report: Respect for Persons, Beneficence, and Justice

The Belmont Report, published in 1979, provides the foundational ethical framework for human subject research in the United States and has influenced ethical guidelines worldwide.

It outlines three fundamental principles:

1. Respect for Persons
    - Recognizing individual autonomy
    - Protecting those with diminished autonomy
2. Beneficence
    - Maximizing benefits and minimizing harm
    - Obligation to protect participants from harm
3. Justice
    - Fair distribution of research benefits and burdens
    - Equal access to the benefits of research

Researchers must:

Declaration of Helsinki: A Global Ethical

Benchmark

The Declaration of Helsinki, first adopted by the World Medical Association in 1964 and regularly updated, serves as a global ethical benchmark for medical research.

Key points include:

1. Primacy of Individual Participants
     - The well-being of the individual research subject takes precedence over all other interests
2. Informed Consent
3. Risk-Benefit Assessment
     - Careful assessment and monitoring of risks and burdens to the research subjects
4. Vulnerable Groups
5. Scientific Requirements and Research Protocols
     - Research must be based on thorough knowledge of scientific literature and other relevant sources of information
6. Research Registration and Publication of Results
7. Use of Placebo
     - Restrictions on the use of placebo when proven interventions exist
8. Post-Trial Provisions
     - Arrangements for post-study access to interventions identified as beneficial

Researchers should:

CIOMS Guidelines: Research in Low-Resource Settings

The Council for International Organizations of Medical Sciences (CIOMS) guidelines provide specific ethical guidance for research in low-resource settings:

1. Responsive Research
   - Research should be responsive to the health needs and priorities of the communities in which it is conducted

2. Fair Participant Selection
   - Equitable selection of study populations to ensure fair distribution of burdens and benefits

3. Community Engagement
   - Active involvement of local communities in research planning and execution

4. Capacity Building

5. Ancillary Care
   - Addressing participants' health needs beyond the scope of the research

6. Post-Trial Access
   - Ensuring continued access to beneficial interventions after the study concludes

7. Fair Benefit Sharing
    - Equitable distribution of the benefits resulting from the research
8. Ethical Review

Researchers working in low-resource settings must:

Ethical Review Committees: Roles and Responsibilities

Ethical Review Committees, also known as Institutional Review Boards (IRBs) or Ethics Committees (ECs), play a crucial role in ensuring the ethical conduct of clinical trials:

1. Protocol Review
    - Comprehensive assessment of research protocols
    - Evaluation of informed consent processes and materials
2. Ongoing Oversight
3. Participant Protection
4. Compliance Monitoring
5. Education and Guidance
6. Documentation and Record-Keeping

Researchers' responsibilities in relation to ERCs include:

ETHICAL CHALLENGES IN VULNERABLE POPULATIONS

Defining Vulnerability in Clinical Research

Vulnerability in clinical research refers to individuals or groups who may be more susceptible to coercion, exploitation, or harm in the research context. Key aspects include:

1. Types of Vulnerability
2. Contextual Nature of Vulnerability
3. Balancing Protection and Inclusion
    - Ensuring adequate protections without unjustly excluding vulnerable groups from research benefits
4. Capacity Assessment
    - Developing and implementing fair and consistent methods for assessing decisional capacity

Researchers must:

Challenges in Pediatric Trials

Pediatric clinical trials present unique ethical challenges:

1. Balancing Protection and Access

- Ensuring children benefit from medical advances while protecting them from research risks
2. Developmental Considerations
3. Informed Consent and Assent
4. Risk Assessment
5. Long-term Follow-up
6. Inclusion of Diverse Pediatric Populations

Strategies for ethical pediatric research include:

Conducting Trials in Pregnant and Lactating Women

Historically underrepresented in clinical research, inclusion of pregnant and lactating women requires careful consideration:

1. Balancing Maternal and Fetal Interests
2. Informed Consent Challenges
3. Pharmacokinetic and Pharmacodynamic Considerations
4. Fetal Safety Monitoring
5. Ethical Justification for Inclusion
6. Lactation Considerations

Researchers should:

Research in Low-Resource Settings

Conducting research in low-resource settings presents unique ethical challenges:

1. Avoiding Exploitation
2. Cultural Sensitivity
3. Informed Consent in Diverse Populations
4. Standard of Care Considerations
5. Post-Trial Access
6. Capacity Building
7. Benefit Sharing

Strategies for ethical research in low-resource settings include:

Trials in Elderly and Cognitively Impaired Populations

Conducting research with elderly and cognitively impaired individuals presents specific ethical challenges:

1. Capacity Assessment
2. Informed Consent Processes
3. Surrogate Decision-Making
4. Risk-Benefit Assessment
5. Inclusion and Representation
6. Privacy and Confidentiality
7. End-of-Life Considerations

Researchers working with these populations should:

- Implement comprehensive capacity assessment protocols
- Develop flexible informed consent processes that accommodate varying levels of cognitive function
- Engage geriatric specialists and experts in cognitive impairment in trial design and oversight
- Implement enhanced safety monitoring and follow-up procedures
- Provide specialized training for research staff on working with elderly and cognitively impaired participants

DIFFERENCES IN CLINICAL TRIAL REGULATIONS GLOBALLY

Harmonization vs. Regional Adaptation: ICH-GCP as a Framework

The International Council for Harmonisation of Technical Requirements for Pharmaceuticals for Human Use (ICH) Good Clinical Practice (GCP) guidelines serve as a global standard for conducting clinical trials.

However, the implementation of these guidelines varies across regions.

1. ICH-GCP Core Principles
2. Regional Adaptations
3. Challenges in Global Harmonization
4. Benefits of Harmonization

Researchers should:

Key Regulatory Differences: Timelines, Documentation, and Inspections

Despite efforts towards harmonization, significant differences exist in regulatory processes across regions:

1. Application and Approval Timelines
2. Documentation Requirements

3. Safety Reporting
4. Inspection Processes
5. Data Requirements

Strategies for managing these differences:

Case Study: Fda Vs. Ema Requirements For A New Drug

To illustrate the differences in regulatory approaches, consider a hypothetical case study of a new drug application:

1. Pre-submission Phase
2. Clinical Trial Application
3. Phase III Trial Design
4. Pediatric Development
5. Accelerated Approval Pathways
6. Marketing Authorization Application
7. Post-approval Requirements

Navigating Multinational Trials: Bridging Data and Approvals

Conducting multinational trials requires careful planning to ensure data acceptability across regions:

1. Early Regulatory Engagement
2. Global Regulatory Strategy
3. Harmonized Protocol Development
4. Addressing Regional Differences in Standard of Care
5. Ethnic Sensitivity Considerations
6. Data Standards and Management
7. Bridging Studies
8. Regulatory Submissions Strategy

Researchers should:

NAVIGATING APPROVALS IN EMERGING MARKETS

Benefits of Conducting Trials in Emerging Markets

Emerging markets offer significant opportunities for clinical research:

1. Large, Treatment-Naïve Populations
2. Cost-Effectiveness
3. Genetic Diversity
4. Addressing Global Health Priorities
5. Market Access
6. Capacity Building

Researchers should carefully evaluate these benefits against potential challenges when planning global trials.

Regulatory Landscape in Asia, Africa, and Latin America

The regulatory environment in emerging markets is diverse and evolving:

1. Asia
2. Africa
3. Latin America

Key considerations:

Fast-Growing Markets: India, China, and Brazil

These markets deserve special attention due to their size and rapid development:

1. India
2. China
3. Brazil

Strategies for success:

Regulatory Bottlenecks and Strategies to Overcome Them

Common challenges in emerging markets include:

1. Lengthy Approval Timelines
    - Strategy: Build in additional time for approvals, consider parallel submissions
2. Evolving Regulatory Requirements
    - Strategy: Maintain close communication with local regulatory experts, monitor for updates

3. Limited Regulatory Capacity
   - Strategy: Provide clear, well-organized submissions, offer to support training initiatives
4. Complex Ethics Committee Processes
   - Strategy: Engage early with local ethics committees, provide comprehensive submission packages
5. Importation Challenges for Study Drugs
   - Strategy: Work with experienced local partners, plan for potential customs delays
6. Data Quality Concerns
   - Strategy: Implement robust training and monitoring programs, consider risk-based approaches
7. Post-Trial Access Issues
   - Strategy: Develop clear plans for continued treatment access, engage with local health authorities

Overcoming these challenges requires:
- Thorough planning and risk assessment
- Flexibility and adaptability in trial design and execution
- Strong local partnerships and on-the-ground presence

- Commitment to capacity building and long-term engagement

ENSURING ETHICAL CONDUCT IN DEVELOPING COUNTRIES

Managing Cultural Sensitivities

Conducting clinical trials in developing countries requires a deep understanding and respect for local cultures:

1. Cultural Competence Training
2. Adapting Communication Styles
3. Respecting Local Hierarchies
4. Gender Considerations
5. Religious and Spiritual Beliefs
6. Family Involvement

Strategies for implementation:

Strengthening Local Ethics Committees

Robust local ethics review is crucial for ensuring the ethical conduct of research:

1. Capacity Building
2. Collaborative Review Processes
3. Infrastructure Support
4. Continuing Education
5. Promoting Independence

6. Enhancing Review Quality

Implementation strategies:

Building Capacity for Ethical and Regulatory Oversight

Long-term improvement in research ethics and regulatory oversight requires systematic capacity building:

1. Training Programs
2. Regulatory Harmonization Efforts
3. Technology Transfer
4. Twinning Programs
5. Research Ethics Centers of Excellence
6. Stakeholder Engagement
7. Sustainable Funding Mechanisms

Implementation approaches:

CASE STUDIES IN MULTI-REGIONAL CLINICAL TRIALS

Case 1: A Global Oncology Trial Across The Us, Eu, And Asia

Scenario: A phase III trial of a novel targeted therapy for advanced lung cancer conducted across 20 countries.
Challenges and Solutions:

1. Regulatory Differences
2. Standard of Care Variations
3. Biomarker Testing
4. Informed Consent
5. Data Management

Key Learnings:

Case 2: A Pediatric Vaccine Trial In Low-Resource Settings

Scenario: A phase III trial of a new vaccine against a tropical disease, conducted primarily in sub-Saharan Africa.

Challenges and Solutions:

1. Ethical Considerations
2. Infrastructure Limitations
3. Follow-up and Retention
4. Adverse Event Reporting
5. Benefit Sharing

Key Learnings:

Case 3: Fast-Tracking Approval In Emerging Markets

Scenario: Seeking rapid approval for a novel diabetes medication in Brazil, Russia, India, and China (BRIC countries).

Challenges and Solutions:

1. Regulatory Strategy
2. Local Clinical Data Requirements
3. Manufacturing and Supply Chain
4. Pricing and Reimbursement
5. Post-Approval Commitments

Key Learnings:

- A flexible, country-specific approach is essential for success in emerging markets
- Early consideration of manufacturing and supply chain issues can prevent delays
- Integrating emerging market strategy into global development plans can accelerate overall timelines

PRACTICAL STRATEGIES FOR MANAGING MULTI-REGIONAL TRIALS

Aligning Regulatory Timelines and Requirements

1. Comprehensive Regulatory Intelligence
2. Integrated Regulatory Strategy
3. Modular Submission Approach
4. Parallel Submissions
5. Regulatory Agency Engagement
6. Flexibility in Clinical Development Plans

Implementation tips:

Preparing for Inspections and Audits

1. Quality Management System
2. Mock Inspections
3. Inspection Readiness Training
4. Central Document Repository
5. Vendor Oversight
6. Data Integrity Measures

7. Communication Plans

Best practices:

Ensuring Ethical Consistency Across Regions

1. Global Ethics Oversight Committee
2. Standardized Ethical Review Process
3. Cultural Competence Training
4. Ethical Issue Escalation Procedure
5. Harmonized Informed Consent Process
6. Consistent Participant Protections
7. Ethical Monitoring and Auditing

Implementation strategies:

Leveraging Technology for Remote Monitoring

1. Risk-Based Monitoring (RBM) Approaches
2. Electronic Data Capture (EDC) Systems
3. Remote Source Data Verification
4. Wearable Devices and Mobile Health Technologies
5. Telemedicine for Patient Assessments
6. Centralized Imaging and ECG Review

7. Artificial Intelligence and Machine Learning

Best practices:

- Ensure all remote monitoring technologies comply with data protection regulations
- Provide comprehensive training for site staff and monitors on remote monitoring tools
- Regularly assess the effectiveness of remote monitoring strategies and adjust as needed

FUTURE OF GLOBAL CLINICAL TRIALS

Decentralized Trials: Ethical and Regulatory Considerations

Decentralized clinical trials (DCTs) are becoming increasingly prevalent, offering new opportunities and challenges:

1. Patient-Centric Trial Design
2. Data Integrity and Security
3. Informed Consent in Virtual Settings
4. Remote Monitoring and Safety Oversight
5. Investigational Product Management
6. Evolving Regulatory Frameworks

Researchers should:

Artificial Intelligence in Clinical Research

AI and machine learning are poised to transform various aspects of clinical trials:

1. Protocol Design and Optimization
2. Patient Matching and Recruitment
3. Real-Time Data Analysis
4. Image Analysis and Diagnostics

5. Natural Language Processing in Adverse Event Reporting
6. Predictive Modeling for Drug Discovery

Researchers must:

Strengthening International Collaboration

Enhanced global cooperation is crucial for advancing clinical research:

1. Harmonization of Data Standards
2. Global Research Networks
3. Collaborative Training Programs
4. Joint Regulatory Initiatives
5. Global Patient Engagement
6. Shared Platforms for Research Transparency
7. Crisis Preparedness and Response

Researchers should:

APPENDICES

Glossary of Regulatory Terms

This glossary provides definitions for key terms commonly used in global clinical trials:

List Of Global Regulatory Authorities

This list includes major regulatory authorities involved in overseeing clinical trials worldwide:

1. United States: Food and Drug Administration (FDA)
2. European Union: European Medicines Agency (EMA)
3. United Kingdom: Medicines and Healthcare products Regulatory Agency (MHRA)
4. Japan: Pharmaceuticals and Medical Devices Agency (PMDA)
5. China: National Medical Products Administration (NMPA)
6. India: Central Drugs Standard Control Organization (CDSCO)
7. Canada: Health Canada
8. Australia: Therapeutic Goods Administration

(TGA)

9. Brazil: Brazilian Health Regulatory Agency (ANVISA)

10. Russia: Ministry of Health of the Russian Federation

11. South Korea: Ministry of Food and Drug Safety (MFDS)

12. Switzerland: Swissmedic

13. Singapore: Health Sciences Authority (HSA)

14. South Africa: South African Health Products Regulatory Authority (SAHPRA)

15. Mexico: Federal Commission for the Protection against Sanitary Risk (COFEPRIS)

References
Key Publications and Guidelines

ABOUT THE AUTHOR

Dr Essam Abdelhakim

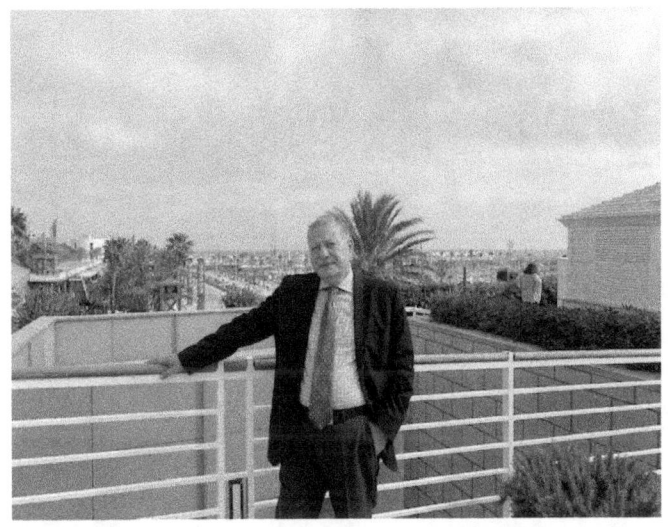

Senior Investigator and Expert in Clinical Research

www.ingramcontent.com/pod-product-compliance
Lightning Source LLC
Chambersburg PA
CBHW070947220526
45471CB00007B/2927